To

Mr. MR Dr. med. Dieter Neumann, Gera
Mr. Dr. med. Jörg Finsterer †, Gera
Mr. Prof. Dr. med. Dirk Eßer, Erfurt

Dr. med. René Keßler

𝔗𝔥𝔢 𝔮𝔲𝔢𝔰𝔱𝔦𝔬𝔫 𝔬𝔣 𝔤𝔲𝔦𝔩𝔱

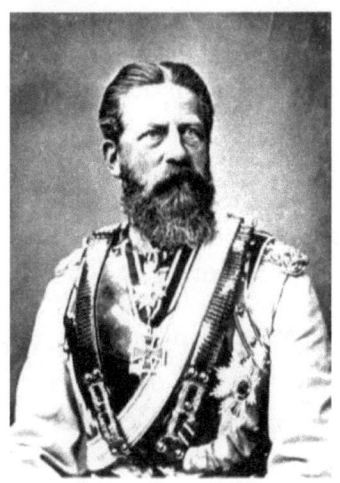

**In the case of the illness of
Emperor Friedrich III (1831-1888)
from an ENT-point of view**

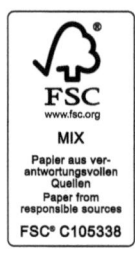

Bibliografische Information der Deutschen Nationalbibliothek:
Die Deutsche Nationalbibliothek verzeichnet diese Publikation in der Deutschen Nationalbibliografie; detaillierte bibliografische Daten sind im Internet über http://dnb.dnb.de abrufbar.

TWENTYSIX – Der Self-Publishing-Verlag
Eine Kooperation zwischen der Verlagsgruppe Random House und BoD – Books on Demand

© 2021 Dr. René Keßler

Herstellung und Verlag:
BoD – Books on Demand, Norderstedt, Germany

ISBN: 978-3740-7805-93

Table of contents

Preamble	p. 7
The story	p. 9
Medical considerations	p. 21
The question of guilt	p. 34
The role of Mackenzie	p. 38
Attempt of a psychological consideration	p. 46
A chain of mistakes and failures	p. 49
Resume	p. 56
The protagonists	p. 57
Literature	p. 62

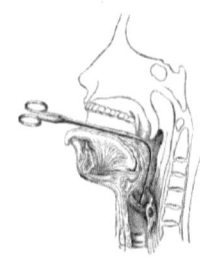
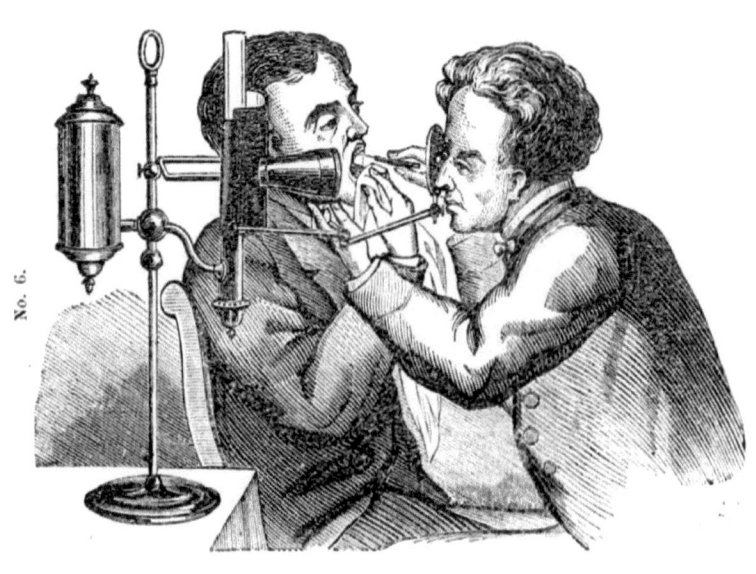

Larynx examination at the time of Friedrich the Third

Preamble

This book looks at the medical history of the German Emperor Friedrich III from the point of view of an ENT doctor. It was important to consider the overall course and not just focus on the role of Mackenzie and Virchow, as it is practised in some sources.

In particular, the primary treatment of the illness and the associated loss of time deserve special attention. In addition, the events must be seen in the context of the medical and technical possibilities of the time, at a time when ENT medicine was still in its infancy. There were still no endoscopes or surgical microscopes and there was a huge uncertainty about the nature of malignant tumors.

Nevertheless, it must be clearly stated that the medical history presents itself as a sequence of treatment errors, misdiagnoses and trench warfare among the treating physicians.

While the Englishman Sir Morell Mackenzie was previously addressed as solely responsible for the emperor's early death from larynx cancer, a more nuanced picture emerges from a critical review of the eyewitness reports and consideration of the medical aspects.

Consequently, it can be considered certain that another doctor, namely Professor Gerhardt, must be regarded as the main culprit. Mackenzie was only called in when the primary therapy had no effect and the tumor was probably already infiltrating the surrounding structures of the larynx. His adherence to the benign nature of the finding was certainly not only based on Virchow's histological results, his personal vanity and lack of self-reflection also contributed significantly to his behavior.

The course of the disease is illustrated by using the reports of the treating physicians and discussed in connection with the respective treatment measures. The subject of discussion is, in addition to the wrong therapeutic decisions and diagnostic omissions, the possibility of further illnesses that could have accelerated the fateful course of the suffering of the crown prince and later emperor.

Dr. med. René Keßler, ENT- doctor, Gera, Germany

In the winter of 2021

The story

Since January 1887, the Prussian heir to the throne Friedrich Wilhelm von Hohenzollern suffered from hoarseness. During a mirror examination on March 6, which was caused by the personal physician Dr. Wegner, the Berlin larynx specialist Professor Gerhardt found a long, pale red, flat nodule (approx. 2x4 mm) on the left vocal cord[1]. Overall, the vocal folds were slightly reddened, but their mobility was intact, which Gerhardt explicitly emphasized in his report[1]. After painful attempts to remove what the Berlin doctor described as primarily benign by means of galva-nocaustic treatments, the 56-year-old Crown Prince could only whisper. The whole procedure of burning off the visible adenoids was not only downright questionable, but very painful, despite the efforts at local anesthesia with cocaine.

Today this "therapy" is hardly understandable any more. But in the spring of 1887, it was used on one of the most important members of the House of Hohenzollern from the end of March to April 7th, almost every day. Gerhardt then stated: "nothing more of this (tumor, author's note) can be seen"[1]. Within four weeks of the prince's cure in

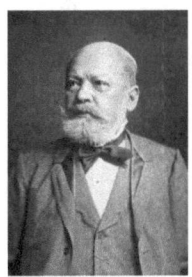

Prof. Gerhardt

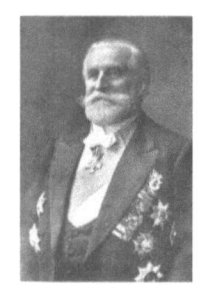

Prof. v. Bergmann

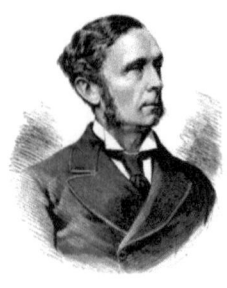

Sir Morell Mackenzie

Bad Ems without an experienced larynx specialist accompanying him, the tumor grew back and the left vocal cord was increasingly restricted in movement.[1]. Gerhardt and the consulted surgeon Ernst von Bergmann made the clinical diagnosis of cancer on May 16 without histological finding and prepared the removal of one side of the larynx (laryngofissure) for May 21st [1]. However, after Bismarck's intervention, Kaiser Wilhelm I forbade the intervention because Friedrich Wilhelm had not given his consent[6]. The Crown Prince was not fully informed about the suspected diagnosis and the associated therapeutic consequences by his first-time practitioners - so the refusal of his consent for an operation that is quite risky is understandable. Bismarck had also recognized this and rightly insinuated that the German doctors wanted "to make the Crown Prince unconscious and to extirpate the larynx without having announced their intention to him"[6].

In Bad Ems, probably at the instigation of a doctor there, the consultation of another larynx specialist was considered. The personal physician Wegner brought the name Morell Mackenzie into play[2;4]. Since 1863 he had a clinic for throat diseases in London and was considered as a proven expert. None of the attending physicians believed that Mackenzie, who was immediately notified, could disagree completely with them. To this day it is unclear what or who prompted Wegner to make this proposal. However, it can be considered certain that Crown Princess Victoria, who came from England being a daughter of the Queen with the same name, bearing in mind her bad experiences with German doctors during the birth of the later Emperor Wilhelm II.

And now begins a chain of peculiarities that still rack the brain of historians and doctors today. After a detailed examination of the patient on May 20, 1887, Mackenzie came to the conclusion that there was no evidence of cancer of the larynx; Friedrich Wilhelm rather suffered from a benign tumor[11]. A tissue sample taken by Mackenzie the following day, consisting of several tiny particles, was given to the German pathologist Virchow for examination. He was the author of the basic work on cellular pathology and pioneer in the field of research into malignant tumors[8]. However, Virchow could not find any cancer and only described irritative changes [1;11].

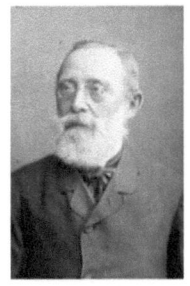

Prof. Virchow

Mackenzie's arrival in Potsdam was the beginning of a partly publicly conducted mud-dinging between him and the German doctors. Encouraged by Virchow's findings, the Englishman continued to interpret the tumor as a benign tumor despite its apparent growth. On June 8, 1887, he performed another intervention on Friedrich Wilhelm and obtained a sample consisting of two pieces of tissue. Virchow referred to this as Pachydermia verrucosa laryngis, a term that is still used today for benign, warty changes in the vocal cords, the first description of which was suggested a few years earlier by Virchow's colleague Juergens (see picture). Although Virchow pointed out in his report that it was not possible to make a clear diagnosis from the material obtained[18], Mackenzie was once again confirmed in his assessment. So he promised the prince that he could cure him without an operation.

To come to the point: the autopsy of the later emperor clearly revealed the diagnosis of larynx cancer. But how could two such excellent people like Mackenzie and Virchow be wrong? This is where the speculation begins. Some dismiss the process as a classic misdiagnosis [7;23], while others use conspiracy theories [15]. Should the heir to the throne, who was considered liberal, be eliminated in order to shake Germany's supremacy on the continent? Or did reactionary circles want to help his son Wilhelm to succeed to the throne early by eliminating the heir to the throne? Shortly after the death of Friedrich III. the allegations of those involved piled up. While the German side, especially Emperor Wilhelm II, accused the Englishman

Mackenzie of the murder of his father[22], the English press accused the German doctors of therapeutic failure by von Bergmann.[15]

Gerhardt himself admitted that there could be the possibility of a malignant tumor at an early stage.[1;2] Additionally, he put Mackenzie in charge of having injured the healthy right vocal cord. Gerhardt increasingly being excluded from the treatment group. He writes in his report that from July 1, 1887, he received no further information about the Crown Prince's illness.

In the meantime the patient's condition deteriorated to such an extent that Mackenzie suggested a new examination, which was carried out in November 1887. After that, the Englishman first expressed his suspicion to the Crown Prince that it might be cancer[1]. A subsequent medical consultation, to which German specialists were also invited, resulted in no consensus on the further procedure apart from mutual allegations and disputes. Although the diagnosis of cancer was generally accepted, the extent of this and thus the therapy remained controversial. Finally, the only option suggested to the Crown Prince was the then extremely risky total larynx removal, the survival rate of which was then less than 10%. But he refused an operation on the grounds that a future emperor without a voice could not fulfill his duties.

After staying in England, Scotland and Venice (and so on), Friedrich Wilhelm finally wanted to find relief from his increasing complaints in the mild climate of San Remo. Friedrich Wilhelm's son, who later became the "World War Emperor" Wilhelm II, indiscreetly and published the cancer diagnosis in the "Reichsanzeiger" on November 15, 1887 without the permission of the doctors. It is also a fact that the aged Wilhelm I, in an order dated from November 17, 1887, bypassing his son, designated his grandson as the de facto successor with the power to sign in the event of his death, but later revised this[12].

By January 1888, the condition of the heir to the throne continued to deteriorate. Fever attacks and persistent pain dominated the picture. Dr. Bramann, von Bergmann's first assistant, was sent to San Remo on the highest orders to be able to perform an immediate tracheotomy as a trained surgeon in an emergency. On January 17th, the patient coughed up a piece of tissue from the larynx. In the histological examination, again carried out by Virchow, one reads a bundle of complicated descriptions and technical terms. The word "cancer" alone does not appear in it [11].

Virchow's successor Professor Waldeyer was convinced that Mackenzie and thus also Virchow acted "against better judgement" and issued false finding[15].

The swelling had meanwhile spread to the right vocal cord and the Crown Prince was only breathing through a narrow, almost invisible gap between the tumor masses. From January onwards, the air emergency reached an increasingly life-threatening extent, so that, in the unanimous opinion of the German doctors present, an incision of the trachea was considered as urgent[1]. Finally Mackenzie also agreed, not without first declining any responsibility[7;13]. On February 9, 1888, Brahmann performed a tracheotomy in San Remo under adverse conditions in the patient's bed. To ensure breathing, the surgeon inserted a silver cannula into the windpipe. After the initial healing tendency, however, increasing breathing problems soon appeared, which led to a "cannula dispute" between the German doctors and Mackenzie. In his monograph "The Illness of Emperor Frederick the Noble", Mackenzie primarily accuses Brahmann and von Bergmann of inserting or incorrectly placing the cannula.

Due to the patient's increasing lung complaints, the internist Kussmaul was sent to San Remo. He also told Mackenzie that it was a throat cancer; He could not find

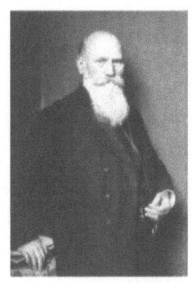

Prof. Waldeyer

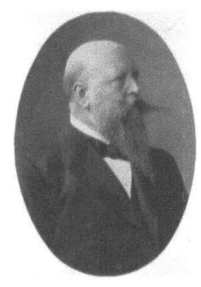

Dr. Bramann

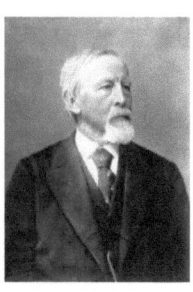

Prof. Kußmaul

evidence of other foci, especially in the lungs[1]. On February 16, 1888, von Bergmann himself believed to have produced fine tissue evidence of the malignancy of the tumor, as he proudly proclaimed in his report. Waldeyer confirmed finding on March 5th[1].

Despite the now obvious misjudgment of the Englishman, Friedrich Wilhelm held on to him. Today it can be taken for granted that his wife, Crown Princess Victoria, played a decisive role in this process[3;4;9;19]. Since the birth of her son, who later became Emperor Wilhelm II, accompanied by medical malpractice, she has shown undisguised distrust of German doctors. The left arm of Wilhelm was damaged as a result of a medical misjudgment during the birth process, which had led to a lifelong disability. Some historians see this flaw and the resulting inferiority complex as the main cause of Wilhelm II's aggressive policies, which ultimately ended in the First World War[14].

Wilhelm I died on March 9, shortly before his 91st birthday. As Emperor, Friedrich Wilhelm took the name Friedrich III. The private feud between Morell Mackenzie and Ernst von Bergmann now entered the final round.
With the active help of the press it had been a dispute between two nations for a long time. Although von Berg-

mann declared to the emperor that he no longer wanted to work with Mackenzie, the majesty did not want to part with his personal physician.

On April 12, von Bergmann had to use a longer cannula in an emergency, which was probably a via falsa (Latin: "wrong way"), here in the sense of incorrect placement of the cannula, which caused damage to the trachea, as Mackenzie stated) (see picture). For the Englishman, the cannula used by von Bergmann was responsible for the further deterioration of the patient's condition[11]. When the emperor expectorated food components from the cannula on June 12, a pharyngeal tube was required to ensure adequate nutrition. The suspicion of a breakthrough of the tumor into the esophagus expressed by the medical council could not be confirmed in the autopsy. Rather, increasing insufficiency of movement of the epiglottis seems to have been responsible for the aspiration of food. Virchow and Waldeyer report about cherry-sized lumps on the base of the epiglottis, which inevitably severely impaired swallowing[1].

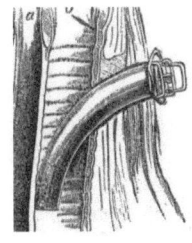

The "german" cannula in the windpipe (from Mackenzie)

Unable to utter even a single sound, keeping communication with little pieces of paper and suffering from the constant painful change of the cannula, the emperor was only a shadow of himself. From the tracheostoma, gummy

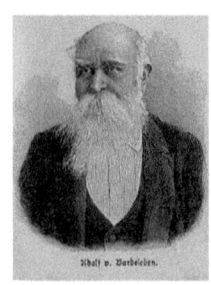

Prof. Bardeleben

fluid drained, which indicated a necrotic dissolution of the tissue. Purulent expectoration, fever and an increasing spread of the tumor to the surrounding skin mark his last days. Professor Bardeleben, who assisted the emperor in the hour of death, reports a high fever and up to 140 breaths per minute[1].

On June 15, Friedrich´s III fate had finally come to an end. He had been on the throne for a full 99 days. Nietzsche saw in his death "a great, decisive misfortune for Germany"[20].

Shortly afterwards Mackenzie rehabilitated himself in front of the German people with a bulletin, which was supposed to prove his innocence in the death of the emperor beyond dispute. The autopsy of the body under the direction of Virchow and Waldeyer revealed an extensive larynx tumor with ingrowth into the trachea and the surrounding structures, regional metastasis in a cervical lymph node and the skin. Friedrich Wilhelm's son Wilhelm ascended the German imperial throne as the second of his name and almost four years later, at the age of 54, Sir Morell Mackenzie died probably of tuberculosis, met with hostility by the Germans, but also by some of his compatriots,. The world maneuvered itself into the First World War. The result is known.

Die Krankheit
Kaiser Friedrich des Dritten

dargestellt

nach amtlichen Quellen

und

den im Königlichen Hausministerium niedergelegten Berichten

der Aerzte

Prof. Bardeleben, Generalarzt I. Kl. und Kgl. Geh. Ober-Med. Rath in Berlin, Prof. von Bergmann, Generalarzt I. Kl. und Geh. Med. Rath in Berlin, Dr. Bramann, erster Assistent der kgl. chirurg. Klinik in Berlin, Prof. Gerhardt, Geh. Med. Rath in Berlin, Prof. Kußmaul, Geheimer Rath in Straßburg i. E., Dr. Landgraf, Stabsarzt in Berlin, Dr. Moritz Schmidt, Sanitätsrath in Frankfurt a. M., Prof. Schrötter, Vorstand der laryngol. Klinik in Wien, Prof. Tobold, Geh. Sanitätsrath in Berlin, Prof. Waldeyer, Geh. Med. Rath in Berlin.

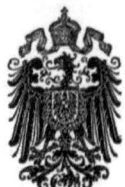

Kaiserl. Reichsdruckerei. Berlin.
1888.

Medical considerations

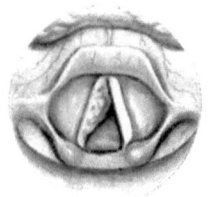

Larynx cancer
(classic exophyte)

From a medical point of view, the death of Friedrich III offers more questions than answers. The primary laryngological examination did not take place until March, although the cardinal symptom hoarseness had been occurring since the beginning of the year. The role played by Friedrich's personal physician, General Doctor Wegner, in this delay has not yet been adequately researched. In any case, there is a first omission in the treatment of the Crown Prince.

The respective descriptions of the tumor deserve particular interest from the perspective of the individual examiner. From the initial inspection by Gerhardt to the first examinations by Mackenzie, the typical picture of a whitish exophyte for vocal cord cancer is never described[1]. This "cauliflower-like" structure on a vocal cord allows the clinical diagnosis of vocal cord cancer with great certainty. (see picture).

Mackenzie's woodcuts provide information about the course of the tumor growth[11]. His first drawing (figure 1) can be reconciled with the clinical picture of a benign polyp. It is therefore quite understandable that he assumed a benign process a priori with the largely smooth surface. Also the other pictures by Mackenzie do not show any typical carcinoma findings (figure 2-5), with the restriction that the larynx was only shown in the so-called "inspiration position" with open vocal folds. The restriction of mobility on the left side, which was described at an early stage, is therefore not understandable. Only the illustration from November 6, 1887 shows that the swelling has spread to the left aryepiglottic fold and the areas under the vocal cord (figure 6).

Malignant tumors of the vocal cords have the lowest rate of metastasis of all carcinomas of the head and neck area[5]. The reason for this is the almost no lymphatic supply and the low proportion of blood vessels. In addition, it is known from clinical experience that many patients survive for several months despite regional metastases.

The engravings from Mackenzie's book "Frederick the Noble and his Doctors" (German edition)

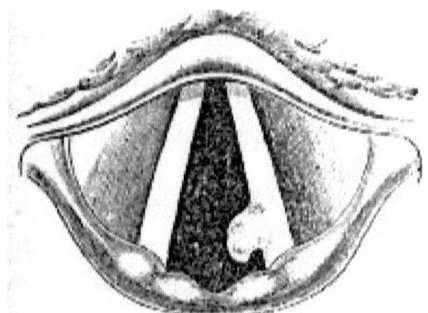

Fig. 1. Skizze des Gewächses, wie dasselbe zuerst aussah.

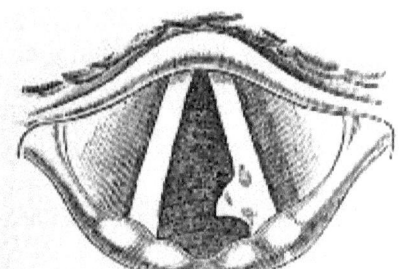

Fig. 2. Skizze des Gewächses nach der ersten Operation. Diese Skizze wurde am 22. Mai angefertigt.

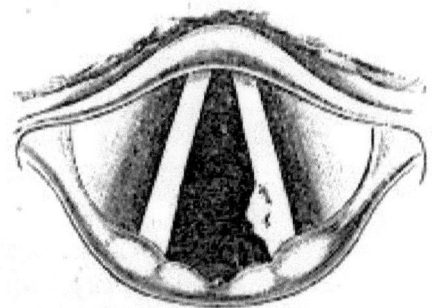

Fig. 3. Skizze des Gewächses nach der dritten Operation.

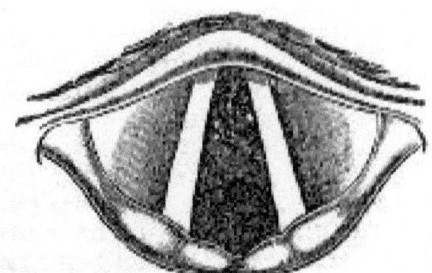

Fig. 4. Skizze, welche am 28. Juni ausgefertigt wurde. Dieselbe zeigt den Kehlkopf nach vollständiger Fortschaffung des Gewächses. Man bemerkt eine sehr geringe Verdickung in der Nähe der rückwärtigen Extremität des linken (im Holzschnitte rechten) Stimmbandes.

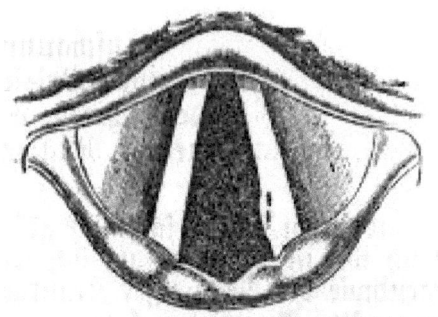

Fig. 5. Skizze, welche Hovell's Beobachtungen am 8. Sept. zeigten.

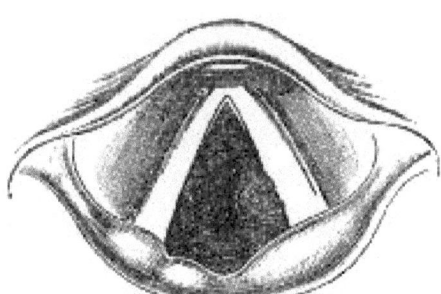

Fig. 6. Eine am 6. Nov. gemachte Skizze, welche ein großes neues Gewächs, einen halben Zoll unterhalb des linken Stimmbandes zeigt und ein kleineres Gewächs unterhalb des rechten Stimmbandes.

The restriction of movement of the left vocal cord, which was already evident in May 1887, allows us to state that the tumor had already exceeded the vocal cord boundaries and had infiltrated surrounding structures such as the cartilage joint.

The statistical survival time for untreated larynx cancer averages twelve months. Infections, bleeding and cachexia are the most common causes of death in addition to suffocation. Distant metastases probably did not exist in the body of the emperor; at least the lungs showed no metastasis. Although the emperor's liver was not explicitly examined, there is no compelling evidence of massive liver metastasis.

Neither edema nor a yellowish discoloration of the sclera, the skin or the mucous membranes are documented in published reports. There was also no intrusion into the large neck vessels, as Virchow and Waldeyer confirm in the autopsy report[1].

The increasing physical exhaustion of the emperor in the course of the illness was described in a flowery manner in almost all reports, but only a very limited consequence was derived from it. The focus of the therapeutic procedure was always on the larynx disease. Only Kussmaul was consulted as an internist to assess the lungs.

In a time without X-ray machines or even sonography and tomography, many findings could not be made by doctors, but the omission of regular full-body examinations is not excusable. So it remains to be seen whether additional illnesses or even secondary cancers have accelerated the course of the disease. However, there are some indications for this.

- The cancer of the vocal cords metastasized slowly. According to the current TNM classification, the later emperor was a T4N1M0 event. Organ failure due to distant metastases cannot be proven.

- As long as breathing can be maintained (by tracheotomy), no larger vessels are affected and no distant metastases are effective, there is no acute danger to life even with larger tumors of the glottis.

- Larynx cancer leads to physical decline relatively late in otherwise healthy middle-aged people. However, a clear reduction in the general condition of the Crown Prince was already documented in the reports of autumn 1887. It cannot be ruled out that infectious, cardiovascular or metabolic diseases have accelerated this.

- In 1886, Friedrich had suffered from measles as Crown Prince. There are various sources. His librarian, for example, is said to have noticed "his whole organism (the Crown Prince, author's note) appeared weak, exhausted and limp[25].

- For a longer period of time, the emperor received pain relievers, which at that time could not be described as fully developed and which had a variety of side effects.

- The cannula changes very likely led to a via falsa, which caused inflammation of the surrounding structures and, as a result, exhaustion of the physical reserves.

- Classical risk factors are hardly described. Although the emperor was known as a pipe smoker, there is no evidence of excessive alcohol consumption as a further predisposing factor for throat cancer.

- A familial burden for cancer, in particular larynx cancer, is not proven in the Hohenzollern house; on the contrary, most of the Hohenzollern princes were considered to be quite stable in terms of health well into old age (Friedrich Wilhelm's father reached the age of

90, his son Wilhelm II over 80 years. Since the Great Elector, the ruling Hohenzollers have been on average 68 years old). However, the son of Friedrich III, Prince Heinrich (1862-1929) also suffered from throat cancer, but reached an age of 66 years.

- It cannot be ruled out that Friedrich contracted an "amorous disease" during a stay in Egypt in 1869 when the Suez Canal was opened. The Frenchman Jean de Bonnefon (1866-1929) drops corresponding hints in his book "Ce` qu on ne peut dive à Berlin" (English:" What one shouldn't say in Berlin "). Mackenzie also informed a friend that the Crown Prince and later emperor had been a "paralytic"[24] - at that time a paraphrase for a syphilis disease. If Friedrich was infected with it, mercury might have been used (secretly?) as a therapeutic agent at that time, which could well lead to physical decline.

The last point deserves special attention. Should Friedrich actually be infected with syphilis in 1869, this venereal disease could have been in the 4th stage at the beginning of his larynx disease in early 1887, where e.g. neurological and psychological symptoms occur.

Medicine agrees that the spirochetes, bacteria that cause syphilis, cannot only through by passed on sexual intercourse, but for instance also through kissing. The incubation period is ten to 90 days, but symptoms of the 1st stage appear on average after two to three weeks.

At the respective entry port (genital part, throat, anus) a small, firm ulcer is found, which is accompanied by the swelling of the surrounding lymph nodes. This heals spontaneously after four to six weeks, and the disease can pass into the second stage. This is followed by the third stage, which is characterized by the appearance of so-called "gums", necrotizing ulcers. And finally the fourth stage follows after about ten to twenty years. The main characteristic of this stage is the involvement of the nervous system. Meningitis, damage to the peripheral nerves or numbness and dizziness are the main symptoms. As a result of this progression of the syphilis, personality changes, epilepsy or depression can occur[27].

Was Friedrich depressed? Did he suffer from personality changes? These questions cannot be answered with certainty. His fatalism ("Learn to suffer without complaining!") and his tolerance could be interpreted as possible clues. However, there are a few important points that are an obstacle to a syphilis infection of the Crown Prince/emperor:

- There are no indications of syphilitic symptoms in the years 1869-1887, in particular not of a primary effect, lymph node swellings or gums. One might argue that such things, if they had been noticed, would have been very delicate and would certainly have been treated like a state secret, but given the large number of doctors involved, they might have come to light in some way, under certain circumstances perhaps only after the emperor's death.

- In Friedrich's wife Victoria, no symptoms are documented that would indicate an (inevitable) infection with syphilis.

- After 1869, Friedrich and his wife had two more daughters (Sophie * 1870; Margarethe * 1872). Neither of the two had the classic signs of congenital syphilis, such as saddle nose, deafness, "barrel teeth".

- And one aspect must not be forgotten either. There is the possibility of the healing of the infection, particularly in the early stages. In literature, this rate is given with more than 30%[27]. So of course this option should also be considered with Friedrich.

If one takes the information from Bardeleben's records and the autopsy report, the most likely cause of death is fatal bronchopneumonia due to aspiration of food and saliva. It is speculative whether this infection could have been prevented through regular tracheal toilet, physical measures or a more optimal cannula.

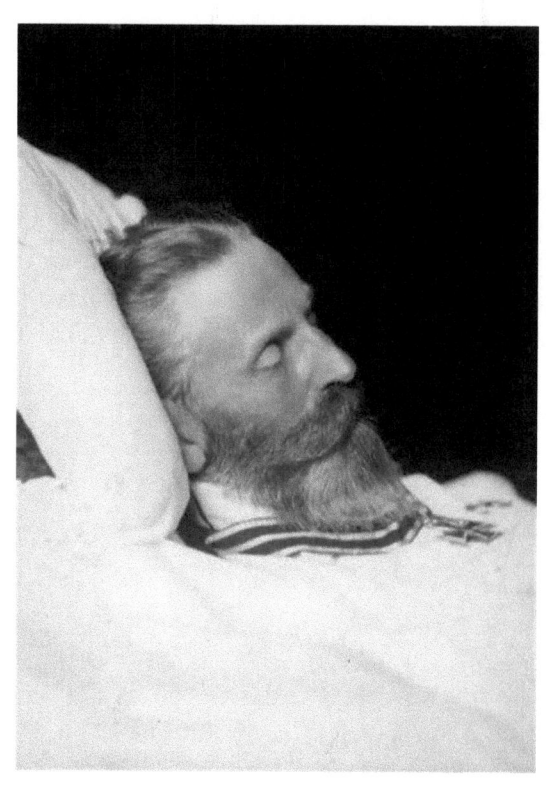

Emperor Friedrich the Third on his death bed

The question of guilt

Till today the German side is unison of the opinion that the main culprit for the death of Friedrich III is the Englishman Mackenzie. A sober observation, however, creates a different picture. The German laryngologist Gerhardt was the first person treating the disease. The open question is why he did not take a single histological preparation during the many operations. Gerhardt himself writes that he was primarily unable to remove the tumor with pliers or ring knife[1]. Then he tried to remove it with a glowing platinum loop in a total of 14 sessions (!). Why were so many "treatments" necessary for a relatively small tumor?

Gerhardt's statements that he no longer saw the tumor on April 8, 1889, but already had concerns about its nature at the beginning of this month, remain contradictory[1]. Why did he not deduce any consequences from this and let weeks pass? With a person like the former Crown Prince in particular, the entire repertoire of medical diagnostics including the histological confirmation of findings would have been indicated and also achievable as early as possible.

The German doctors, including Gerhardt, accused Mackenzie of insisting on histological facts, but they themselves only relied on clinical appearance. From this, however, a fundamental question arises: Why did they not try to substantiate the clinical suspicion with a representative histology before Mackenzie's appearance?

Or was Mackenzie right when he accused Gerhardt in his justification of not being able to use the laryngeal forceps? This would of course imply the impossibility of a representative tissue removal. From March 6 until Mackenzie's arrival on May 20, 1887, Gerhardt had ample opportunity to make a reliable diagnosis or to seek advice from a (German) specialist colleague. It would certainly have been easy to consult Schrötter, Tobold, Schmidt or only other leading German laryngologists at this time.

In this context it must be mentioned that already in 1886 the doctor Bernhard Fränkel (1836-1911) from Berlin reported on a transoral removal of a small carcinoma of the vocal cords[16]. Couldn't he, as an experienced doctor, have been involved in the treatment of the Crown Prince? And why didn't Gerhardt accompany the Crown Prince to Bad Ems? There he would have been able to get an idea of the further course every day and, if necessary, intervene earlier. Why, in contrast to Mackenzie, did he not produce any pictorial representations of the findings? With all these considerations one must always keep in mind that the patient was the heir to the throne of the German Empire and thus neither economic nor logistical obstacles can be used as an excuse for the omissions mentioned.

It was only when the tumor had grown significantly that Gerhardt decided to even consider the possibility of consulting another specialist. In retrospect, he must have been extremely happy that Mackenzie did the treatment for him. His reference that from May 1887 onwards he had not learned anything more about the further course therefore appears more as a cry of relief than regret.

Another fact that has been largely ignored so far in the literature is that the then leading laryngeal surgeon Prof. Billroth (1829-1894) from Vienna, who had already performed the first total larynx removal in 1873, was not involved. Prof. Bergmann's experience in the field of larynx surgery was certainly far behind that of Billroth. Was it vanity or personal resentment that prevented Gerhardt, Bergmann and others from consulting the great Viennese surgeon?

To sum up the above, Gerhardt must be blamed for the emperor's early death. Clear failures, such as his renouncement of histological verification and discontinuous control of the findings, coupled with uncertainty and at least a questionable primary treatment, set the course for the further fateful course. In addition, there was a lack of self-criticism and a lack of patient education. If Gerhardt had tried to make a histological diagnosis right at the beginning of the treatment and had fully informed the Crown Prince in time about the scope of the event, Mackenzie, who was brought in later, would hardly have been able to support his benignity hypothesis for so long.

The role of Mackenzie

The appointment of the English laryngologist as treating physician is always ascribed to the Crown Princess Victoria in historiography. However, there is no conclusive evidence for this. The actual suggestion came from the personal physician Dr. Wegner. Whether he wanted to please the Crown Princess or even received the order from her can only be speculated. Laryngologists Stoerk from Vienna and Rauchfuß from Petersburg were also in discussion. In any case, the doctors present, Gerhardt, von Bergmann and Wegner, agreed on Mackenzie, who was notified by telegram and arrived in Berlin on May 20, 1887.

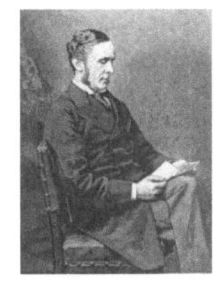

Sir Morell Mackenzie

In his book "Friedrich the Noble and His Doctors", Mackenzie comments on the first meeting with Gerhardt and von Bergmann. He attests Gerhardt only having average knowledge of throat diseases, but he explains about von Bergmann that his name is not mentioned in the laryngological literature, which clearly (and correctly) means that he has almost had no experience in the laryngological field.

At the same time, Mackenzie expresses his astonishment that apart from Prof. Tobold („among the current generation of doctors" he is hardly more than nominis umbra) (English: "shadow", author's note) no other German specialist was called in. However, he did not give names. Even at this introductory point in his writing, Mackenzie succeeds in creating a fundamental doubt in the reader about the professional competence of his colleagues. In the case of Prof. Tobold, however, he was wrong. For decades he had been an expert in the field of laryngology, a pioneer in larynx diagnostics and the author of a standard work on laryngoscopy.

The German doctors around von Bergmann wanted to perform a half-sided larynx resection as early as May 1887. In the run-up to the planned splitting of the larynx, there was no express consent of the Crown Prince, which prompted Bismarck to raise an objection and to inform Emperor Wilhelm I, the father of Friedrich. who then forbade carrying out the operation without his son's consent[6]. The failure to provide the patient with comprehensive information about the findings and the planned intervention was clearly due to Gerhardt and von Bergmann, which is often forgotten in the follow-up reviews. The fact that the operation did not take place later was due to Mackenzie's intervention. He fundamentally questioned the usefulness of a larynx operation and drew attention to the dangers that he considered life-threatening, as he explained in his justification[11]. In a meticulously executed statistic, Mackenzie pointed to a high mortality rate (27.2 percent) and a high risk of recurrence (54.5 percent) after the laryngofissure (split larynx) inaugurated by the consultant.

From a purely medicolegal point of view, Mackenzie acted correctly from today's perspective by speaking out against an operation on May 20, 1887 due to the lack of histological evidence of cancer and with reference to possible complications. The criticism of Gerhardt and especially of von Bergmann that he focused too much on the histological diagnosis of Virchow and neglected the clinical appearance is ill-considered.

Mackenzie did the right thing by attempting a biopsy and looking at Virchow's findings. In all later discussions it is not assessed that the tissue removal by Mackenzie was done on a vocal cord that had been operated 14 times by Gerhardt. Even under today's modern conditions and with the use of the surgical microscope, cancerous tissue cannot always be detected, which often requires re-biopsies. Mackenzie is to be blamed for ignoring Virchow's warning to infer from just on piece of tissue findings about the entire disease and made at least four more frustrating attempts to remove the tumor in the following weeks.

But how did Mackenzie manage to assert himself as a personal physician? It has certainly not been hidden from the Crown Prince that his suffering was progressing despite the promise of healing that Mackenzie regularly made. On the one hand, he uttered the legendary saying to his son "Learn to suffer without complaining!" as a sign of Prussian hardship. On the other hand, he wept in his wife's arms at the fears that plagued him about their future[7].

The planning of the larynx operation by Gerhardt and von Bergmann in May 1887 without his consent may have, if not destroyed, at least shaken his trust in German doctors. In doing so, a basic principle of therapeutic action, namely the education of the patient, was violated. The Crown Princess certainly played a role in the course of treatment that should not be underestimated. According to various sources, she was never able to make friends with the diagnosis of cancer and the associated consequences and almost hysterically clung to Mackenzie and his conviction that the diagnosis was benign[3;19]. In addition, she did nothing to make the full scope of the disease clear to herself and her husband at an early stage. From her experiences as an English-born Crown Princess, she was rather hostile to everything German. In particular, she criticized the lack of art and science at German courts[4]. Mackenzie's engaging personality and his charming demeanor did the rest to make him preferred to the somewhat stiff German professors, who were all civil servants.

The main reason for her aversion to the German doctors, however, is to be found in the birth of her first child, who later became Emperor Wilhelm II. This was done by the German gynecologist Professor Martin. The birth process turned out to be extremely difficult because the child was in the breech position. Forcibly turning the left arm caused a nerve lesion on the infant's arm plexus.

This not only affected the development and usability of the arm for life; even in his childhood and youth, Wilhelm had to endure many painful and senseless "attempts at therapy"[14]. From the summation of these aspects, it seems natural that Victoria should stand by her compatriot. In view of the undoubtedly existing emotional closeness of the imperial couple, which is not exactly typical of ruling marriages, she also had a correspondingly large influence on her husband's decisions. Even though Mackenzie's appointment to the medical team was probably not initiated by her, the Crown Princess is to be regarded as decisive for his stay.

In considering the literature, Sir Morell Mackenzie appears to be solely responsible for the emperor's quick death[7;23]. This statement, mostly fed by the German side, is not only undifferentiated. It is wrong. Mackenzie was undoubtedly an expert in laryngology. He had extensive knowledge in the field of laryngeal diseases, which is evident not least from his bibliography. His standard work "The diseases of the throat and nose" was also translated into German. But as a "safety physician" he was pathologically conscious of his reputation. Several reports document that before potentially dangerous even minor operations in connection with the treatment of Friedrich Wilhelm he always pointed out that he could not take over any responsibility.

He did not even want to be responsible for the tracheotomy, as it is clearly expressed in Bramann's notes. Strictly speaking, in his therapeutic strategy he adhered to the rule "No dangerous operation without reliable histology!", which was by no means binding at the time when pathology was pioneer work. In addition, an early correction of his diagnosis would have jeopardized his reputation and also the reputation to the Crown Princess.

It should also not be forgotten that Sir Morell Mackenzie did not have an equal opponent with the German surgeon von Bergmann, whom he probably disliked from the start due to his lack of knowledge of laryngology. He was also strengthened in his inviolable role by his patient himself, who awarded him the house order of the Hohenzollern on the occasion of the emperor's coronation and appointed him imperial personal physician.

Mackenzie's meticulousness in the description of the course of the disease should be emphasized, illustrated by six woodcuts of the findings, which document the development of the tumor from April 20 to November 6, 1887. The other laryngologists were content in their justifications with verbose explanations of the findings.

The fact is: From today's point of view, Mackenzie is most likely to be accused of subordinating the clinical appearance of the tumor to the histological diagnosis of Virchow and only admitting the possibility of suffering from cancer in November 1887. It remains unclear why this was revoked by him on January 7, 1888 in the British Medical Journal[17].

He enjoyed the emperor's full trust until the end, perhaps also because he showed his patient more empathy than the other doctors. Despite some polemical statements about his German colleagues, his work "Friedrich the Noble and his Doctors" can be considered exemplary for the exact documentation of a medical history.

Attempt of a psychological consideration

Even for a psychological layman, a fundamental question arises in view of the drama surrounding Friedrich's illness: How was Mackenzie able to assert himself against the "superior power" of German doctors from the start?

From a formal point of view, the Englishman had a not inconsiderable reputation, not at least because of the laryngological standard work he had written, but the large number of his opponents alone should have developed a persuasive power in the patient, e.g. an early operation (larynx splitting) would have been made possible.

This only allows the conclusion that Mackenzie was far superior to the German doctors in terms of empathy, but also in his self-portrayal. In addition, the influence of Crown Princess Victoria, who must undoubtedly have been a patron of Mackenzie, on the entire procedure receives too little attention in most pieces of literature or is viewed too one-sidedly[25].

All sources agree that Victoria and Friedrich cultivated an intimate relationship, which was almost unusual in the circles of the nobility at the time. For this reason, a significant influence of the princess on her husband is

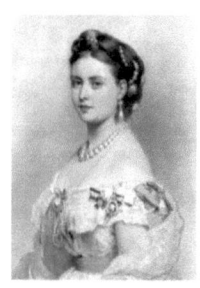
Kaiserin Victoria

obvious. Her resentment towards the German doctors undoubtedly contributed to "swearing" the Crown Prince and later Emperor to Mackenzie's opinion.

At the same time it seems strange that Friedrich showed himself to be almost completely resistant to the opinion of von Bergmann and the other German doctors and still allowed a regular examination by these doctors without being contradicted. In other words: the German doctors were allowed to examine the crown prince and later emperor but not treat them.

Another point should be discussed in this context. Perhaps Mackenzie was right when he said that e.g. Gerhardt had no exceptional knowledge and von Bergmann had little experience in the field of larynx diseases. Medicine is, per se, a science of experience, and the doctor gains experience primarily through working with the patient. A lack of experience not only leads to misjudgments and incorrect therapy, it also implies a lack of practice. Perhaps the German doctors were not as adept as the English with regard to the examination technique of the larynx, which was then still in its infancy. And maybe Mackenzie was just softer and more empathetic in his approach. Which patient does not prefer a doctor who can examine and treat gently and painlessly?

In recognition of this complex situation, it is hardly surprising that Mackenzie was able to maintain his prominent position with the crown Prince/ emperor over the entire period.

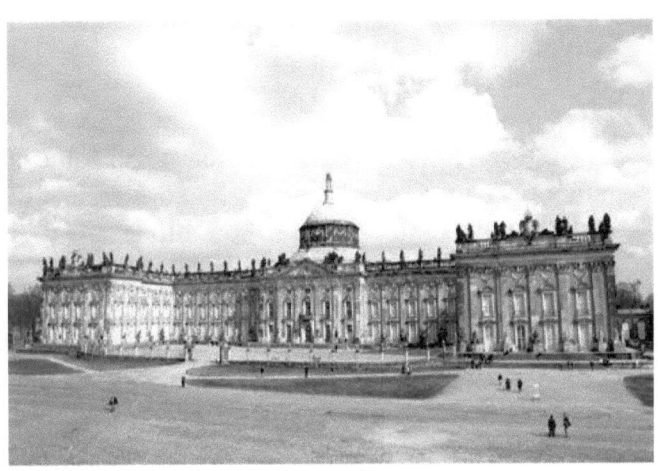

The new Palace in Potsdam – Friedrich the Third died here

A chain of mistakes and failures

The emperor's medical history can be seen as a continuous chain of wrong decisions and treatments:

1. The belated diagnosis - at least two months passed between the initial symptoms and the first laryngological examination.

2. The procedures with the platinum loop - in the spring of 1887, Gerhardt carried out a total of 14 attempts to remove the left vocal cord almost daily. Even under the difficult conditions of indirect laryngoscopy at the time, the tumor should have been eliminated after one or two interventions. It is also not clear to today's observer why Gerhardt opted for this method and why, above all, he did not obtain any usable histology.

3. Gerhardt's compulsion to have confidants - although Gerhardt commented early on in his reports about the probable malignancy of the ulcer and also von Bergman was convinced of it, they

gratefully allowed Mackenzie to be consulted by Wegner in harmony with the Crown Princess. Wouldn't it have been more advisable if they had consistently defended their suspicions without "safeguarding" anyone and had let the Crown Prince into their therapy plan in good time?

4. The histological specimens - Virchow is commonly assumed to have been misdiagnosed. From the reports of those involved, however, it is clear that von Mackenzie only examined tiny particles from a vocal cord that had been operated on several times before. It should be clear to everyone that they did not necessarily lead to a reliable diagnosis. A submucous growth of the cancer (under the mucous membrane) must also be discussed, which was not shown in the samples taken at the beginning. Even under today's conditions, such findings can often only be seen through imaging diagnostics (e.g. MRI). Despite the best efforts, these "occult" carcinomas cannot be confirmed with a biopsy, since the tissue is only removed from the upper, healthy layers. Only as the process progresses are these infiltrated by the

cancer cells, making the diagnosis histologically verifiable. In this context, Virchow's cautious statement must be seen, who warned against drawing uncritical conclusions about the entire clinical picture from his examination results.

5. The lack of communication between the German doctors and the patient - if it is true that a few hours before the planned larynx split on May 20, 1887, the Crown Prince had no idea of the impending operation and therefore his consent was not available. Here Gerhardt and the entire council can be blamed. How little was generally known about the scope of the Crown Prince's illness is made clear by the fact that non-medical professionals such as Bismarck and Emperor Wilhelm I were able to intervene successfully.

6. Mackenzie's behavior - that Mackenzie did not recognize the true character of the tumor during his first examination is surprising but not impossible based on his great clinical experience. In addition, he was a cautious man who, according to his doctrine, did not want to cause complications

through an operation without a clear histology. From today's perspective, he acted correctly. The only reproach is that he did not support his hypothesis with a new biopsy and did not correctly interpret the growth of the tumor. In addition, as the protégé of the Crown Princess, he found himself in a moral dilemma, bearing in mind her strict denial of the possible malignancy of the tumor. If he had agreed to the originally planned operation (split larynx) and the cancer had not been confirmed or the patient would have died during the operation, the trust of the Crown Princess and the entire ruling house would have been used up.

7. The interference of Bismarck and the emperor - as with all high-ranking personalities, in this case too, non-medical professionals felt called upon to express their opinion without being clear about possible consequences. This interference was favored by the civil servant status of the German doctors, who were thus receiving orders in the hierarchical system and could only act independently to a limited extent.

8. The patient's indulgence - the patience of Friedrich Wilhelm is absolutely incomprehensible. Starting with Gerhardt's painful attempts to remove the ulcer to the rather brutal change of cannulas shortly before his death, nothing has been passed on of the patient's rebellion. Although the dispute between the doctors and their insecurity should not have escaped him, he never spoke a word of power or even called a new team of doctors. For a man who distinguished himself in several battles through commitment and decisiveness, this wait-and-see behavior was rather untypical. One plausible explanation can only be that he was largely left in the dark about his illness. This is undoubtedly supported by the larynx operation, inaugurated without his consent, which was only prevented by imperial intervention and Mackenzie's appearance.

Another, albeit unlikely, possibility is the presence of a psychiatric illness of the Crown Prince, e.g. caused by an infection with syphilis. Its late stage, neurosyphilis, is linked by a decline in intelligence and perceptual disorders.

9. The cowardice of von Bergmann - although full professor at the first German surgical clinic at the Charité in Berlin, von Bergmann was not a recognized expert on throat diseases. He was certainly flattered by the trust of the Crown Prince which he initially placed in the matter. But he was not able to justify this trust, because he wanted to split the larynx without the patient's consent and information. Compared to Mackenzie, he was at a disadvantage from the start because of his lack of knowledge of laryngology.

10. The so-called "many cooks spoil the porridge syndrome". Why have over 20 doctors been consulted without any changes in treatment strategy? At the same time, however, it seems shameful that an assistant doctor, Bramann, had to perform the tracheostomy in San Remo under unworthy conditions. The discontinuous check of findings is also noticeable, especially during the Crown Prince's stay in Bad Ems and during his trips to England, Scotland and Italy.

11. The disregard of the accompanying symptoms - apart from Kussmaul, no other internist of rank was called in to assess the patient. The treatment focused almost exclusively on the larynx. From today's perspective, it must also be noted critically that, if one studies the reports of the treating physicians, the trachea was apparently never aspirated after the tracheotomy or any physiotherapeutic measures (expectorant inhalations, etc.) were not used. Perhaps this could have delayed the development and course of the ultimately fatal pneumonia. In addition, according to the statements of the medical bulletins, no attention was paid to the patient's other organ systems, which is unacceptable in view of the increasing physical decline of the patient.

Resumè

The example of Emperor Friedrich III. shows how medical inconsistency, personal quarrels and a lack of transparency put the patient's life and health at risk, and how the pursuit of an alleged reputation coupled with therapeutic failures led to the patient's painful death. The decisive factor in the course, however, was the approach taken by the first treating physician, namely Professor Gerhards. His hesitant attitude and questionable primary treatment along with a lack of patient education have largely determined the course of the disease.

The widespread picture that sees Mackenzie as the main culprit must therefore be contradicted. It remains to be speculated whether the emperor could have been saved by an early operation. The complications that were not manageable at that time and the associated high death rate speak against it. It remains unclear whether additional diseases, such as an infectious or metabolic disease, had a negative impact on the course, although some evidence imply it.

The protagonists

According to the sources, over 20 doctors were involved in the treatment. The most important are:

Prof. Dr. Heinrich Adolf von Bardeleben (1819-1895), Privy Chief Medical Officer, surgeon, treated the emperor during his last days, ennobled in 1891

Prof. Dr. Ernst Gustav Benjamin von Bergmann (1836-1907), Privy Medical Councilor, surgeon, in the medical council since May 1887, advocated an early cancer acceptance and an operation, but was unable to assert himself against Mackenzie

Dr. Friedrich Gustav von Bramann (1854-1913), assistant doctor to von Bergmann, performed the tracheotomy under primitive conditions, later professor in Halle, ennobled by Wilhelm II in 1890

Prof. Dr. Carl Jakob Adolf Christian Gerhardt (1833-1902), Secret Medical Councilor, internist and one of the leading German laryngologists, carried out the galvanoscaustic treatments at the Crown Prince, and after its failure, he represented the cancer hypothesis without drawing the necessary conclusions in time, his influence on the treatment was almost completely stopped after Mackenzie was called in

Prof. Dr. Leopold Anton Dismas Schrötter von Kristelli (1837-1908), internist and laryngologist from Vienna, was appointed to San Remo in November 1887, informed the Crown Prince of the diagnosis and pleaded for a laryngeal removal

Prof. Dr. Carl Philipp Adolf Konrad Kussmaul (1822-1902), Privy Councilor, internist and polymath, prepared an internal and pulmonary report, according to which cancer of the larynx was the only cause of the Crown Prince's disease

Dr. Wilhelm Landgraf, Medical Officer, Gerhardt's assistant, accompanied the Crown Prince to England in the summer of 1887, and made Mackenzie aware of the progression of the disease

Dr. Gustav Adolph von Lauer (1808-1889), General Doctor, personal physician to Kaiser Wilhelm I, only active in an advisory capacity

Prof. Dr. Ernst Viktor von Leyden (1832-1910), internist and cancer specialist, active in an advisory capacity; there is no medical report from him

Sir Morell Mackenzie (1837-1892), English laryngologist, author of various works on throat diseases, ran one of the first specialist clinics in London; was consulted for treatment from April 1887, considered the tumor to be benign for a long time, not only because of the lack of evidence of histology, and, not least because of its influence at court, prevented extensive operations, ennobled by Queen Victoria in 1888

Dr. Johann Friedrich Moritz Schmidt-Metzler (1838-1907), Secret Medical Councilor, laryngologist from Frankfurt/ M., represented cancer hypothesis from November 1887, but also made a "contagious" disease responsible (allusion to a possible sexually transmitted disease)

Prof. Dr. Adelbert Tobold (1827-1907), Secret Medical Councilor, surgeon and laryngologist, author of the "Textbook of Laryngoscopy" (Berlin 1863), was already convinced of the malignancy of the tumor during the first examination in 1887 and pleaded for a quick operation, later withdrew and advocated a full larynx removal

Prof. Dr. Rudolf Ludwig Karl Virchow (1821-1902), Privy Councilor, pathologist and founder of the theory of cellular pathology, as a member of the German Liberal Party, member of the German Reichstag, enemy of Bismarck; for a long time could not find any definite malignancy in the tissue samples, but warned against generalizing this and carried out the dissection of the corpse together with Prof. Waldeyer

Prof. Dr. Heinrich Wilhelm von Waldeyer-Hartz (1836-1921), anatomist and pathologist, director of the anatomical institute, was the first to determine cancer in the histological specimen, Virchow's critic, with whom he carried out the dissection of the corpse, later ennobled

Dr. August von Wegner (1846-1905), General Doctor, personal physician of the crown prince and of the later emperor, did not consult the laryngologist Gerhardt until March, at his suggestion Mackenzie was entrusted with the treatment, ennobled by Friedrich III.

Literature

(1) Die Krankheit Kaiser Friedrich III. dargestellt nach amtlichen Quellen den im königlichen Hausministerium niedergelegten Berichten der Ärzte, Kaiserliche Reichsdruckerei, Berlin 1888

(2) Amtspresse Preußens, VII. Jahrgang. No. 68. Neueste Mittheilungen. Verantwortlicher Herausgeber: Dr. H. Klee. Berlin 1888.

(3) Arden, Dorothee.: Kronprinzessin Victoria Kaiserin Friedrich, Magisterarbeit Frankfurt a.M. 2000,

(4) Aufermann, Marie Luise.: Der persönliche Anteil der Kaiserin Friedrich an der deutschen Politik, Inaugural-Dissertation zur Erlangung der Doktorwürde der Hohen Philosophischen und Naturwissenschaftlichen Fakultät der Westfälischen Wilhelms-Universität zu Münster i.W., 1932 (Berufung Mackenzies, Rolle der Kaiserin)

(5) Becker, Walter; Naumann, Hans Heinz; Pfaltz, Carl Rudolf: Hals-Nasen-Ohren-Heilkunde, Stuttgart 1986

(6) Bismarck, Otto Fürst v.: Gedanken und Erinnerungen. hrsgb. von Horst Kohl, 1. u. 2. Bd., Stuttgart 1928.

(7) Freund, Michael.: Das Drama der 99 Tage, Krankheit und Tod Friedrichs III:, Köln/Berlin 1966

(8) Hauptmann, Steffen; Schnalke, T.: Rudolf Virchows Sicht der malignen Geschwülste, Pathologe 2001, 22:291–295

(9) Hessen, Rainer von (Hg), Victoria Kaiserin Friedrich, Campus-Verlag Frankfurt/M. 2002

(10) Mann, Golo: Deutsche Geschichte des 19. und 20. Jahrhunderts, Büchergilde Gutenberg, Frankfurt am Main 1958, S. 483 (Charakter Friedrichs)

(11) Mackenzie, Morell: Friedrich der Edle und seine Ärzte, Styrum und Leipzig 1888

(12)　　Neugebauer Wolfgang (Hg.), Handbuch der preußischen Geschichte, Band III, Berlin 2000

(13)　　N.N., Der Spiegel Nr. 21/1967, S. 76-79

(14)　　Röhl, John C.G.: Wilhelm II., München 1993

(15)　　Vandenberg, Philipp.: Die heimlichen Herrscher, München 1991, S. 107-148

(16)　　Werner, Jochen A., Engenhart-Cabillic, Rita: Kehlkopfkrebs – Diagnostik und Therapie im Wandel der Zeit, Ärzteblatt Hessen 9/2005, S. 122-127

(17)　　http://www.hno-marburg.de/

(18)　　https://www.innominatesociety.com/

(19)　　https://www.kaiserinfriedrich.de/

(20)　　https://www.preussenchronik.de/

(21)　　https://www.uniklinik-ulm.de/

(22) https://www.wikipedia.de/

(23) Zehmisch, Heinz: Die Kehlkopferkrankung bei Kaiser Friedrich III., Ärzteblatt Sachsen 6/2003, S. 226 (Mackenzie alleinschuldig, ein englischer Doktor tötete meinen Vater)

(24) Dr. Mackenzies Geheimnis, Der Spiegel 19/1947

(25) Freund, Michael: Das Drama der 99 Tage, Kiepenheuer & Witsch, Köln-Berlin, 1966

(26) Wolf, H.-J.: Die Krankheit Friedrich III. und ihre Wirkung auf die deutsche und englische Öffentlichkeit, Berliner Medizinisch Verlagsanstalt, Berlin-Lichterfelde, 1958

(27) Nasemann, Th., Sauerbrey, W: Lehrbuch der Hautkrankheiten und vernerischen Infektionen, Springer-Verlag, 1987

Illustrations

Fig. 1-6 und picture p. 18:

Mackenzie, Morell: Friedrich der Edle und seine Ärzte, Styrum und Leipzig, 1888

picture p. 12 "Pachydermia laryngis"
picture p. 21 "larynx cancer"

von Eicken, Carl; Schulz van Treek, A.: Atlas der Hals-Nasen-Ohren-Krankheiten, Thieme Stuttgart, 1951

picture p. 22

Packard, Francis R.: Diseases of the Nose, Throat and Ear, London, 1909

All other pictures: https://www.wikipedia.de/

Thanks to my beloved wife and to my children.

Many thanks go to Christina Martens for the translation and to Ilona Frank for the useful notes.